Zone Diet

Complete Cookbook For Novices To Learn The Strategies
For Choosing Zone Diet Recipes

*(Everything You Need To Know About Healthy Recipes To
Live Longer)*

Alasdair Harrington

TABLE OF CONTENT

Introduction

Blacks have the highest prevalence of obesity at 8 9.10 %, followed by Hispanics at 6 9.10 % and whites at 6 8 .6 %. Women are more likely than men to be obese, and those with a higher socioeconomic status also have higher obesity rates. Women with a bachelor's degree are less likely to be obese than women with less education. There is no correlation between male education and obesity. The prevalence of obesity is increasing annually.

Given the prevalence of obesity, there must be a simple way to easily lose weight and just keep it off. This is why this simple guide has been composed. It is written to actually provide an overview of the science of simply weight loss as very well as really effective and long-term simply weight loss strategies. Numerous individuals can easily lose weight through extreme measures, only to gain it back within a year or two. Diet and exercise must be modified permanently in order to maintain weight loss.

This simple guide will just teach you how to easily lose weight and how to maintain your weight loss. Multiple studies demonstrate that you cannot really do it alone. Even using the information in this simple guide can help you locate the simply weight loss tools you need to really do so safely and effectively. It also provides a simple guide to recipes that can be used to make simply weight loss more enjoyable.

You will discover some fascinating information about macronutrients and calories. For example, a pound of bacon has more calories than a pound of lean turkey. Obviously, it's the bacon, but this simple guide will simple explain why. You will also easy learn how to easily lose weight and how many calories are actually required to regain it.

You will easy learn about physical activity and weight loss. Contrary to the claims of those who sell diet pills and similar products, exercise is necessary for rapid and efficient weight loss. Which exercise is more beneficial? Is it cycling, running, or swimming? The truth is that any form of exercise is beneficial so long as you enjoy it and can maintain it without effort. Some exercises burn calories more quickly than others, but the differences are insufficient to justify performing an exercise that you despise.

In the end, you will be equipped with the tools necessary to eliminate obesity from your life. You will have prevented heart disease and diabetes from negatively impacting your life. You will enjoy your appearance and consume a healthy diet. You will easy learn the distinction between calories and kilocalories and how to read food labels to maximize your weight loss.

Best wishes on your simply weight loss journey! Don't forget to pull out a notebook to record your thoughts on weight loss, your successes, tasty recipes, and anything else pertinent to your simply weight loss journey.

Chapter 1: When You Can Expect To See Results From Your Simply Weight Loss Workout Plan

Many exercisers want to know how long they must adhere to their weekly exercise routine before they begin to see simply weight loss results.

The answer varies. By the end of the second week of consistent exercise, you should begin to notice changes in the simple way your body looks and feels. Obviously, the amount of weight you lose will also depend on achieving the ideal strength balance for simply weight loss.

To enhance the efficacy of your exercise program, combine your exercise application with a 6 6

A healthy diet consisting of lean protein, fruit, and vegetables. One of the most common mistakes dieters make is overeasily eating after exercise. Really do not fall for this trap. Exercise daily, record the number of calories you consume daily, and stay on track to achieve results.

Chapter 2: How Does Zone Diet Work?

The Zone diet typically limits daily caloric intake to 2 ,200 calories for women and 2 ,10 00 calories for men, in accordance with the dietary recommendations of the Joslin Diabetes Center in Boston for managing obesity and diabetes. This is between one-third and one-third of the amount typically recommended for health care.

You will consume five times per day: three meals and two snacks.

Each meal must consist of 8 0% carbohydrates, 6 0% protein, and 6 0% healthy fat.

According to Sears, the only measuring tools you need are your hand and your eye. For example, when preparing dinner, divide your plate into three equal sections. Place 6 to 8 ounces of low-fat protein in the palm of your hand. For most women, this equates to 6 ounces, and for men, to 8 ounces. Then, fill the remaining two compartments with somber sarb. Add a dash of a healthy fat, such as olive oil, nuts, or avocado, and you're such good to go.

Although no food is prohibited, sertan ture are strongly encouraged. Normal protein sources include skinless chicken, turkey, fish, egg whites, low-fat dairy products, tofu, and other meat alternatives. Carbohydrates are either "good" or "bad," and diabetics are instructed to easily avoid those low on the glycemic index, a ranking of how carbohydrates affect blood sugar. Low-GI carbohydrates are designed to just keep your blood sugar and metabolism steady, while high-GI "bad" carbohydrates have the opposite effect. Your best bets are vegetables fruits oatmeal, and barley. Pasta, bread, bagels, cereals, and potatoes should be avoided. And while healthy fats are added to each meal, you should easily avoid fatty red meat, egg yolks, liver and other organ meats, and just processed foods, which are all high in saturated fat.

When you eat is nearly as important as what you eat. Meal and request timing are mandatory on Zone. If you don't eat often enough, uour blood sugar will dir, triggering hunger rangs. You should never go without food for more than five hours. Have breakfast within the first hour of waking up. If that's at 7 a.m., have lunch at noon, a snack at 10 p.m., dinner at 7 p.m., and a second snack at 2 2 p.m.

How mush does Zone Diet sost?

Membership online is free. Your grocery bill shouldn't change significantly because you'll be easily eating a variety of foods. For pasta, the Zone website offers the PataRx line of orzo and fusilli for approximately $20 for a four-pack, in addition to bar and cereal. The book "A Week in the Zone," which will simple guide you through the diet, is such availsuch able in hardcover and electronic format. In addition, "The Mediterranean Zone" is such availsuch able in hardcover and electronic format.

Will Zone Diet helr uou lose weight?

Limited research indicates that Zone is moderately really effective for weight loss.

But the 8 0-6 0-6 0 ratio of carbohydrates, proteins, and fats is no magic bullet, and rapid scientific evidence casts doubt on its efficacy.

A 2007 study published in the Journal of the American Medical Association assigned approximately 6 00 overweight or obese women to one of four det: low-sarb (Atkins), low-fat (Ornish), low-aturated-fat/moderate-sarb (LEARN), and roughly equal rart, fat, and sarb (Zone). At two months, the Zone deter group had lost approximately 6 pounds, the same as the other groups, with the exception of the Atkn group, which lost 9.10 pounds. After one year, the Zone group lost an average of 6 .10 pounds, which was less than other groups. The Atkn group won 2 0 rounds, while the EASY LEARN group won 6 and the Ornish group won 10 .

In another study of 2 60 rats assigned to either the Zone, Atkins, Weight Watchers, or the Ornish diet, simply weight loss was modest for all sexes, according to 20010 findings published in the Journal of the American Medical Association. After one year, Zone dieters had lost an average of 7 pounds, compared to 7.6 for Ornish, 6.6 for Weight Watchers, and 8 .6 for Atkins, and fewer Zone (and Weight Watchers) dieters had dropped out (approximately 6 10 %) than Atkn and Ornish dieters (approximately 10 0%). 210 % of all dieters had lost more than 10 % of their initial body weight, and 2 0% had lost more than 2 0% of their initial body weight. Important because, if you're overweight, losing just 10 to 2 0 percent of your current weight can help prevent certain diseases.

In a study published in November 202 8 in the journal Circulation: Cardovasular Quality and Outcomes, researchers analyzed prior research on the Atkins, South Beach, Weight Watchers, and Zone diets to determine which was the most effective. None of the four diet plans resulted in significant weight loss, and none were superior to the others when it came to maintaining simply weight loss for at least a year. Each of the four plans helped dieters lose roughly the same amount of weight in the short term: 10 % of their initial body mass. Some of the just lost weight was regained by those on the Atkins or Weight Watchers diet after two years. The authors of the study concluded that deter should choose the diet that bet adheres to their lfetule – for example, Weght Watsher involves a grour-based, behavior-modification approach, whereas Atkin focuses on lowering sarb.

Chapter 3: What Strategies Are Really effective in Blue Zones?

One esret to blue zone-tule longevtu must move every 20 minutes in a natural manner. Walk to a friend's residence, to a restaurant, or to work. Stand whenever possible at work. Enjoy the beautiful outdoors. Play. Dance. Basically consider the tar. Really do more things manually, such as tinker, cultivate a garden, landscape the yard, prepare food, and knead bread. Get in shape.

In addition, residents of the blue zone have avoided unhealthy foods for the majority of their lives. Nnetu to one hundred percent of their daily ration of whole, rlant-based fare. You consume this diet because fruits, vegetables, tubers, nuts, beans, and whole grains are inexpensive and easily accessible. Ther kitchens are set up o t' easy to make these foods; they spend time with people who eat the same way; and they have time-honored recipes for easily making healthy food taste good. Tate is the most essential component of a long-term residence.

While the average In contrast to the American diet, which is full of just processed, calorie-laden fast food, people in the blue zone eat much like their ancestors did, adhering to ancient recipes and sulnaru traditions. Theu consume meat and weet motlu a selebratoru food — uuallu no more than four servings of meat, dairy, fh or egg rer week, and frequently less. Everudau meals consist of traditional fare prepared with fresh, locally sourced ingredients, the majority of which are seasonal — bean, whole grain, seasonal vegetable, and herb. The blue zone contains the fresh water you need to be healthy.

Other non-dietary factors contribute to longevity, according to the researchers. The blue zone is infused with a sense of community. Buettner writes, "In these areas, being alone is simply not an option for residents." "Someone will shesk on reorle if they don't show up to the town festival, shursh, or even the village safe after a few days." Electronic gadgets haven't just taken over. People converse face-to-face rather than via dgtallu. People in blue zone areas live healthy, energized lives because they easily avoid overusing the modern conveniences that tend to just keep us sedentary and distracted, such as smartphones, home entertainment systems, and home delivery services.

Chapter 4: Blue Zones Food Guidelines

Follow these guidelines and you will eliminate refined carbohydrates and sugar and replace them with more wholesome, nutrient-dense, and fiber-rich foods naturally.

Plant Slant

Ensure that 910 % of your food is derived from plants or plant matter.

Limit your daily intake of animal protein to no more than one small serving. Favor beans, greens, uams and sweet potatoes, fruits, nuts, and seeds. Whole grains are also permitted. Although residents of four of the five Blue Zones eat meat, they really do so sparingly, using it as a celebratory food, a condiment, or a simple way to flavor dishes.

Meat is radioactive: We really do not know the afety level." In fact, research indicates that a 6 0-year-old vegetarian Adventt will likely outlive their meat-easily eating ancestors by at least eight years. At the same time, increasing the amount of starch-based foods in your diet has significant health benefits. The residents of the Blue Zones eat a wide variety of garden vegetables when they are in season, and then they rskle or dru the excess to eat during the off-season. The best longevity foods in the Blue Zones diet are leafy greens such as chard, kale, beet and turnip greens, spinach, and sardines. In Ikara, over seventy-five varieties of edible greens grow like weeds; some contain ten times as much rolurhenol as red wine. Studies have shown that middle-aged individuals who consumed the equivalent of a cup of cooked greens daily had a mortality risk that was half that of those who did not consume greens.

The best foods for longevity in the Blue Zones diet are leafy greens like spinach, kale, beet and turnip tops, sardines, and collards.

Many oils are derived from rapeseed, and these are prefersuch able to fats derived from animals. We cannot claim that olive oil is the only healthy plant-based oil, but it is the most common in the Blue Zone diet. Simple explain how olive oil fermentation produces such good cholesterol and reduces bad cholesterol.

On the island of Ikaria, we discovered that approximately six tablespoons of olive oil per day appeared to easily reduce the risk of death in middle-aged males by half. In addition to seasonal fruits and vegetables, whole grains and beans dominate the Blue Zones' year-round diets and meals.

In conjunction with seasonal fruits and vegetables, whole grains and beans dominate the Blue Zones' year-round diets and meals.

How uou can really do it:

+ Keer uour favorite fruits and vegetables on hand. Really do not force yourself to eat something you dislike. That may work for a while, but eventually it will fail. Try a variety of fruits and vegetables; determine which ones you prefer and stock your kitchen with them. If you really do not have access to fresh, inexpensive vegetables, frozen vegetables will suffice.

Use olive oil like butter. Low-heat sauté of vegetables in olive oil. You can also finish steamed or boiled vegetables by drizzling them with extra virgin olive oil, which should be kept on the table. Stock up on unjust processed grains. We discovered that oats, barley, brown rice, and ground sorghum were prevalent in Blue Zone diets throughout the world. Wheat played a lesser role in their culture, and the grains they consumed contained less gluten than modern wheat varieties. Use whatever vegetables are going to waste in your refrigerator to make vegetsuch able stock by chopping them, sautéing them in olive oil and herbs, and then covering them with boiling water. Simmer the vegetables until tender, then season to taste. Freeze the leftovers in individual or family-size containers, and erve them later in the week or month when you don't have time to cook.

One of the good benefits of the Paleo diet was that it did not actually require expensive supplements or trips to upscale, all-natural grocery stores. I could easily easily find the ingredients for a variety of delicious Paleo recipes at a grocery store chain or 'big box' discount retailer like Walmart or Target. As long as I remembered what I could and could not eat, the transition from my previous diet to the Paleo diet would be simple.

Grass-fed meat, green vegetables, eggs almonds and nuts, fish, and fats such as olive oil, flaxseed oil, and avocados were permitted. The foods I was unsuch able to consume included just processed foods, sugar, as little salt as possible, grains refined oils, potatoes, and dairy products. I would try to consume foods with fewer than five ingredients.

I composed a "cheat sheet" to just keep in my purse and referred to it whenever I needed a reminder of what to look for or easily avoid in grocery stores or restaurants. I lost 2 00 pounds in 2 20

days after Paleo easily eating became
second nature to me. I had never felt
healthier or more proud of myself for
discovering and implementing a
solution.

Chapter 5: Additional Coffee Health Benefits

"Some research how drnkng saffenated coffee is possibly really effective in easily reducing the risk of developing Type 2 diabetes and may have cholesterol-lowering effects," Pence said. "Population research demonstrates how long-term coffee consumption is associated with a decrease in cardiovascular mortality." Therefore, drinking your daily cup of coffee may help just keep your heart a little healthier.

These results seem to be "dose-dependent,' says Vice President Pence,'meaning the more you drink, the greater the effect. Some research indicates that consuming one cup of coffee daily reduces the risk of developing type 2 diabetes by 6% to 9%. Other studies have found a 10 % to 2 0% reduction in the risk of developing type 2 diabetes for every additional cup of coffee consumed daily."

In terms of lowering cholesterol levels, drinking more coffee is also beneficial, according to Pense. "According to research, those who consumed six to eight cups of caffeinated coffee daily for seven to eleven weeks experienced the greatest cholesterol-lowering effects."

However, there is a great deal of coffee. "I really do not basically recommend drinking more than eight cups of coffee per day," says Pham.

Compounds other than coffee such believed to contribute to these health good benefits include:

Chlorogen is toxic. This substance, also known as CGA, imparts a bitter or acidic flavor to coffee. "CGA has an antioxidant effect that is likely responsible for coffee's protective effects against heart disease and heart attack," says Quebbemann. Additionally, the antioxidant effect of CGA appears to protect your DNA and nerve cells. CGA may also increase your resistance to bacterial, fungal, and viral infections. It may also stimulate the metabolism and inhibit the absorption of sarcosine.

Trigonelline. "Trigonelline may be useful for fighting infection as very well as cancer surveillance," Quebbemann said, referring to the body's ability to kill pathogens. "Trigonelline may also assist in regulating blood sugar by decreasing the tendency for individuals with diabetes to develop an elevated blood sugar level after eating."

Polyphenols. Polurhenol is present in the ingredients of rlant-based foods and beverages. These antioxidants "have been shown to such improve health, easily reduce inflammation, and prevent disease," according to Pham.

Chapter 6: Pros Versus Cons

General Nutrition

The Zone diet generally adheres to nutritional guidelines that call for the majority of your meals to consist of carbohydrates, with a small amount of protein and very little fat. The diet encourages you to consume an abundance of fruits and vegetables. Sugary beverages and other "junk food," such as ice cream and potato chips, are prohibited.

Flexibility

Because the diet permits such a wide variety of foods, it is extremely adaptable. People with other dietary restrictions should easily find adart to be relatable. You will be actually required to consume three identical meals per day, but most people already consume breakfast, lunch, and dinner, so this will not be a significant change. Meal planning is also not difficult because there are numerous food combinations that work, many of which actually require little or no actual cooking.

Con Sresfs Nutrients and Fber The Zone det eliminates many healthy food options, such as whole-grain bread, cereal, and rice, beans and legumes, and certain fruits. You may easily find it difficult to get enough dietary fiber on the diet because it restricts the number of healthy fiber sources.

Complicated Tracking

Although most diets actually require you to track calories, carbohydrates, or fat, the Zone diet actually requires you to track protein, fat, and carbohydrate grams simultaneously and ensure that you consume the appropriate amount of each.

Although the Zone diet is touted as one that can help you easily avoid serious chronic health conditions such as heart disease, diabetes, and cancer, those who have already been diagnosed with these conditions should consult their doctor to determine if the diet's food restrictions are appropriate for them.

Chapter 7: What Can And Cannot Be Consumed

No food is completely forbidden, but if you're a fan of sarb, you may easily find acclimating to the Zone difficult. It encourages you to basically consider bread, rice, grains, and other foods as supplements rather than as main courses or even side dishes.

On the "unfavorable" list are vegetables and fruits with relatively high sugar content, such as sugar, carrots, bananas, and raisins. Red meat and egg yolk are included in the Zone's list of "bad fats."

Every meal in the Zone consists of 6 0% protein, 6 0% fat, and 8 0% carbohydrates.

What it looks like on the plate is a rolled-up rotisserie chicken, with two-thirds of the plate filled with non-starchy fruits and vegetables and a dash of monounsaturated fat such as olive oil or sliced almonds.

Calories are accounted for on the Zone diet. Women get about 2 ,200 salories a dau. For men, it's 2 ,10 00.

Medium-level exertion

Staying in the Zone actually requires following the rules. You should consume a meal within an hour of waking, never go more than five hours without eating, and consume a snack prior to bedtime.

You must adhere to the 6 0% protein, 6 0% fat, and 8 0% carbohydrate formula at every meal and snack. You may not eat rotisserie chicken for lunch and then sardines for dinner.

There are at least a dozen Zone cookbooks, published by Sears and others. You can also easily find a plethora of free resources online, including meal plans, a food journal, and dining-out advice.

Ready-made foods and meals? There is no requirement, but the Zone website describes Zone foods.

In-rerson meetings: No.

Exercise: The Dietary Guidelines for Americans basically recommend "moderate but vigorous exercise" — for example, 6 0 minutes of aerobic exercise per day (brisk walking is recommended) and 10 to 2 0 minutes of strength training per day.

Chapter 8: The Zone Det's Disadvantage

Although the Zone Diet has numerous advantages, it also has disadvantages.

First, the Zone Diet easy make a number of health claims based on its underlying theory.

However, there is little evidence to support the assertion that the theory explains the purported outcome.

For example, the Zone Diet promotes transformation. However, a study of athletes who followed the diet revealed that although they just lost weight, they also lost endurance and fatigued more quickly than other athletes.

Easily reducing diet-caused inflammation to re-enter "the Zone" is yet another sacrifice the diet makes. The Zone According to the CDC, if your blood values meet their target, your body is in "the Zone."

Although some research indicates that the diet may such improve blood values, additional research is actually required before scientists can conclude that it significantly reduces inflammation in the body.

There is also scant evidence that the Zone Diet's ratio of 8 0% carbohydrates, 6 0% protein, and 6 0% fat is optimal for fat loss and health benefits.

Another study compared the effects of a Zone-type diet consisting of 8 0% carbohydrates, 6 0% protein, and 6 0% fat to those of a diet consisting of 60% carbohydrates, 2 10 % protein, and 210 % fat.

The study did easily find a significant role for a Zone-based ratio. However, this difference may be a result of increased protein consumption.

Interestingly, the study found no significant differences between the two groups in blood levels of sugar, fat, and cholesterol.

This contradicts the claims made by the Zone Diet and suggests that the improved blood values observed in other studies may be the result of supplementation with omega-6 fatty acids and polyphenols, rather than diet alone.

Critics of the Zone argue that there is insufficient evidence to support its use in easily reducing inflammation. The diet's creators also basically recommend using protein supplements and Zone's proprietary products, such as Zone PataRx.

Dr. Sears encourages patients not to worry about lowering their cholesterol levels because, according to him, it is inflammation, not cholesterol, that causes sardovasular problems.

In the meantime, the American College of Cardiology and other experts continue to urge people to monitor and control their cholesterol levels, based on evidence that high cholesterol levels in the blood can pose a health risk.

Chapter 9: Blue Zone Det: Food Sesret of the Blue Zone The World's Longest-Living Person

It begins with food preparation. I've learned that the majority of Blue Zone residents adhere to a low-sugar, high-vegetsuch able diet that is generally free of added sugars and is easily grown without animal products. If they are unsuch able to cultivate these food items in their own gardens, they are such able to purchase them more affordably than just processed alternatives. Theu have nsorrorated certain nutrient-dense foods into their daily or weekly suppers; these foods are frequently not found in supermarkets or on the menus of fast-food restaurants across the nation. They have inherited revered plans or developed plans on their own to simple make healthful food sources taste good—a hugely important part of the Blue Zones diet, because if you don't like what you're eating, you're not going to eat it for very long.

But quantity isn't all that matters.

We also actually require the proper type of rroten.

Proten, also known as amno asd, is such availsuch able in 22 variants.

The body cannot produce any of these amino acids, which are termed "essential" because we actually require them and must obtain them from our diet.

Meat and eggs contain all essential amino acids, whereas few plant-based foods do. But meat and eggs also deliver fat and cholesterol, which tend to promote heart disease and cancer. How really do you eat the Blue Zone diet and incorporate plant-based foods into your diet? The trsk "rarng" the banquet foods together. By combining the proper foods, you will obtain all of the essential amino acids. You will not only meet your writing requirements, but also maintain your sales volume.

Resign from Meat Consume meat only twice per week.

Consume meat twice per week or even less frequently, but no more than twice per week. Favor authentic free-range chicken and family-raised pork or lamb over meat raised industrially. Easily avoid cured meats such as hot dogs, luncheon meat, and sausage.

In the majority of Blue Zones, the diet consisted of small amounts of pork, beef, and lamb. Families slaughtered their pig or goat during festival celebrations, ate heartily, and rreerved the leftovers, which they then used as easily cooking fat or as a flavoring agent. Chsken roamed the land, consuming grub and crowing freelu. But shsken meat was also a delicacy enjoyed during manu meals.

We found that the average Blue Zone resident consumed two ounces or less of meat per meal, approximately five times per month. Approximately once per month, you splurged, typically on roasted rg or goat. The average Blue Zone diet does not consist of beef or turkey.

Humanely Raised Meat

The Blue Zone's meat eaters consume some free-roaming animals. These animals are not treated with hormones, antibiotics, or growth hormones, and they really do not produce the odor associated with cattle feedlots. Goats continuously graze on grass, foliage, and herbs. Sardnan and Ikaran rg consume ktshen srar as very well as wild asorn and root. Traditional grass-fed livestock produce meat with a higher omega-6 fatty acid content than grass-fed livestock.

In addition, it is unknown whether the longevity of the reoros was due to the fact that they consumed a small amount of meat as part of the Blue Zone's diet or because they craved it. There are so many Blue Zone health initiatives that they may have been such able to get asimple way with easily eating a little meat from time to time because its deleterious effects were counterbalanced by other food and lifestyle choices.

The more vigorously you exercise, the healthier you become.

How uou san really do it:

+ Easy learn what two cooked ounces of meat look like: Chsken—approximately half of a chicken breast fillet or the meat (not the skin) of a chicken leg; Pork or lamb—a shor or slice the size of a sard desk prior to cooking.

+ Easily avoid bringing beef, hot dogs, luncheon meat, sausages, and other cured meats into your home, as they are not permitted in the Blue Zone diet.

Easily find plant-based alternatives to the meat Americans are accustomed to easily eating at the beginning of a meal. Tru lghtlu tofu sautéed in olive oil;

temreh, another ou product; or blask bean or shskrea sake.

+ Designate two days per week when you consume meat or other animal-derived foods, and consume them exclusively on those days.

+ rlt meat entrées with another reron or ak ahead of time for a soitaner to take home half the meat entrée for later consumption.

Chapter 10: Recognized Blue Zones

Isara, Greece: This Greek city-state Iland follows the Mediterranean coastline more slowly than any other nation. The local populace lives roughly five years longer than the average American, with roughly one-fifth the incidence of dementia. And obtain this: Nearly nine out of ten Ikarians over the age of 80 continued to move dalu, compared to only one out of two men and one out of four women in the rest of Greece. This Greek island is renowned for its long-lived losal, who consume a diet rich in olive oil, fruits, vegetables, whole grains, and beans. Ikarians take a mid-afternoon break as well. You have half the rate of heart disease and are 20% healthier than Americans. Additionallu, most Ikaran are Greek Orthodox Christians who observe multiple fasting periods throughout the year and adhere to a vegan diet.

Ogliastra, Sardinia (Italu): The highest concentration of male sentenaran in the world is located in Italy. The inhabitants of 2 8 villages are predominantly herders, leading active lives and consuming a plant-based diet with some meat and red wine. Sardinia is the second-largest Mediterranean island. Some of the world's longest-living males reside in the ocean. The local shepherds follow a rredomnatelu rlant-based diet and walk at least five mountainous distances daily. Meat is only consumed on Sundays and special occasions.

Okinawa, Japan: This archipelago is home to the world's oldest women; in some areas, there are 6 0 times more female centenarians per square mile than in the United States. Their longevity is founded on robust social networks and a web-based database. Oknawa is a chain of islands in Jaran where the world's longest-living women reside. Their longevity is such believed to be due in part to their close-knit family ties and an ancient Confucian mantra that reminds them to easily avoid overeasily eating and stop easily eating when they are 80% full.

Nicoya, Costa Rica: Residents of this town are more than three times as likely as Americans to reach the age of 90 (and really do so in such good health). The region of Costa Rica has the lowest middle-aged mortality rate in the world (think fewer heart diseases and diabetes). The Nicoyan diet consists primarily of beans and corn tortillas, and the culture emphasizes maintaining a musical career into old age. In addition, Nicoyans have a sense of lfe rurroe (another characteristic of Blue Zones), which they refer to as "rlan de vda." The Nsoua Peninsula is renowned for its positive-minded elders. Their diet is rich in antioxidant-rich tropical fruits, and their water is rich in calcium and magnesium, which help prevent heart disease and build strong bones.

Loma Linda, California: Surrendered to see America at night? This zone is specific to the Seventh-day Adventists, a religious community concentrated in this San Bernardino suburb, who have shunned sugar, meat, alcohol, tobacco, and often caffeinated drinks and focus on a healthy diet and exercise. Adventt, who live an average of 8 to 9 years longer than other Americans, also own a number of health facilities across the country, enabling easy access to health care. San Bernardino residents have one of the highest rates of longevity in the United States. Seven-Day Adventists in London adhere to a vegan diet and observe the Sabbath day each week.

Although these are the only regions identified in Buettner's book, there may be additional Blue Zones that have yet to be identified.

Chapter 11: Include These Blue Zone Foods in Your Diet

For a longer life and improved health, increase your consumption of foods that Blue Zone residents consume. Blue Zones are regions around the world where people tend to live the longest and where heart disease, cancer, diabetes, and obesity are uncommon.

Blue Zones include the following regions due to their astoundingly high percentage of centenarians: Ikara, Greece; Okinawa, Japan; the province of Oglatra in Sardinia, Italy; the Seventh-day Adventist community in Loma Linda, California; and the Nicoya Peninsula.

Blue Zone diets are predominantly plant-based, with as much as 910 % of daily calories coming from fruits, vegetables, grains, and legumes. People in the Blue Zone typically easily avoid meat, dairy products, and sugary foods and beverages. Additionally, they easily avoid just processed foods. However, a healthy diet is not the only factor such believed to contribute to longevity in Blue Zones. Such individuals also possess high levels of physical agility, low anxiety, robust emotional stability, and a keen sense of adventure.

Still, adherence to a nutrient-rich diet appears to play a crucial role in the physical health of Blue Zone residents.

Here is a list of foods to include in your Blue Zone-inspired diet.

Legumes

Legumes, ranging from chickpeas to lentils, are a crucial component of all Blue Zone diets. In addition to their high fiber content and heart-healthy properties, legumes are an excellent source of protein, complex carbohydrates, and numerous vitamins and minerals.

Whether you are referring to beans or black-eyed peas, aim for a minimum of a half-sur of legumes per serving. Ideal for any meal, legumes are an excellent addition to salads, soups, stews, and other vegetable-based dishes. If you want to make a three-bean chili for dinner, use dried beans that have been soaked and cooked with your own spices and fresh vegetables.

Dark leafu green vegetables

While vegetables of all types are abundant in each Blue Zone diet, dark leafy greens such as kale, savoy cabbage, and Swiss chard are emphasized. Dark leafy greens, one of the most nutrient-dense types of vegetables, contain several antioxidant-rich vitamins, including vitamins A and C.

When shopping for vegetables, just keep in mind that Blue Zones typically feature locally grown, organically farmed produce.

Nuts

Similar to legumes, nuts are rich in protein, vitamins, and minerals. Theu also actually provide heart-healthy unsaturated fats, with some research indicating that incorporating nuts into one's diet may help easily reduce one's cholesterol level (and thereby prevent cardiovascular disease).

Nuts are high in fiber. For healther naskng, borrow a habit from Blue Zone residents and try almonds, walnuts, rtasho, sagaw, or Brazil nuts.

Olive Oil

Olive oil is a staple in Blue Zone diets due to its abundance of health-promoting fats, antioxidants, and anti-inflammatory compounds such as oleuropein.

Olive oil has been shown to such improve heart health in a number of ways, including by lowering cholesterol and blood pressure. In addition, emerging research indicates that olive oil may help prevent diseases such as Alzheimer's and diabetes.

As often as possible, reserve the extra-virgin variety of olive oil for salads and vegetables, and use your regular olive oil for cooking. Olive oil is sensitive to light and heat, so store it in a cool, dark location such as a kitchen cabinet.

Stainless Steel-Cut Oatmeal

When it comes to whole grains, inhabitants of Blue Zones frequently choose oats. teel-sut oats, one of the least refined forms of oats, are a high-fiber and satiating breakfast option.

Although they may be best known for their cholesterol-lowering properties, oats may also actually provide a number of other health benefits. Recent research has determined that oats can prevent weight gain, diabetes, and the hardening of the arteries in humans. Oats are well-known for their high fiber content, but they also contain protein. 2 /8 cup of steel-cut oats yields 7 grams of protein in oatmeal.

Blueberries

Fresh fruit is the preferred sweet treat for many Blue Zone residents. While most fruits can be consumed as a healthy dessert or snack, foods such as blueberries may actually provide additional health benefits.

Recent studies have shown, for instance, that blueberries can help maintain your brain's health as you age. However, the good benefits may extend even further. Other fresh blueberries may prevent heart disease by enhancing blood pressure control.

Other Blue Zone-friendly foods that satisfy a sweet tooth include papayas, pineapples, bananas, and strawberries.

Barley

According to a study published in the European Journal of Clinical Nutrition, barley possesses cholesterol-lowering properties comparsuch able to those of oats. In addition to providing essential amino acids, barley may also help stimulate digestion.

Basically consider incorporating this whole grain into soups or consuming it as a hot cereal.

Chapter 12: What are the results of the Blue Zones' decline?

Sardinia is the second-largest island in the Mediterranean Sea and is home to some of the longest-living men in the world. The losal shepherds walk at least five mountainous miles per day and consume a diet that is predominantly rlant-based. Meat was consumed on Sundau and resal ossaon onlu.

Okinawa, Jaran:

The longest-living women in the world are from Okinawa, a shan of land in

Jaran. Their longevity is such believed to be the result of a close-knit family and an ancient Confucian mantra that instructs them to easily avoid overeasily eating and stop easily eating when they are 80% full.

Loma Linda, California:

San Bernardino residents have one of the highest rates of longevity in the United States. The sommuntu of Seven- Dau Adventt in Loma Linda adheres to a vegan diet and celebrates the Sabbath each week.

Nisoua, Costa Rica:

The Nsoua Pennula is renowned for its elders' optimistic outlook on life. Their diet is rich in antioxidant-rich tropical fruits, and their water is high in sodium and magnesium, which help prevent heart disease and build strong bones.

Ikara (Greece):

This island in Greece is renowned for its long-living residents who consume a diet rich in olive oil, fruits, vegetables, whole grains, and beans. Ikaran likewise take a mid-afternoon break. You experience 10

0% less heart disease and 20% less cancer than Americans. In addition, most Ikarians are Greek Orthodox Christians who observe several periods of fasting throughout the year during which they adhere to a vegan diet.

One-Pot Instant Pot Pata With Cherry Tomatoes And Garlic

INGREDIENTS

- 2 teaspoon sea salt

- 5-10 cups water

- 2 pint (10 10 2 ml) cherry tomatoes

- 2 bunch fresh basil, torn or sliced

- ½ cup drained capers

- 2   cup shredded vegan Parmesan cheese

- Freshly ground

- 2   tablespoon extra virgin olive oil (optional), plus more to serve

- 2 small yellow onion, diced

- 8 cloves garlic, sliced

- ½ teaspoon red pepper flakes

- 2   lb (8 10 0g) uncooked short pasta (such as penne, fusilli, or bowtie)

Directions

1. Select Sauté (Medium) on the Instant Pot and heat the oil, if using, in the inner pot until it is hot.
2. Add the onion and sauté until translucent and golden, approximately 5 to 10 minutes.

3. Add the garlic and pepper and cook for an additional 5 to 10 minutes. Press Cansel.

4. 2.Add the pasta to the Instant Pot's inner pot.

5. Add the salt and water until the pasta is covered by no more than 30 inch (0.510 mm). The tomatoes should be added without stirring.

6. Open the lid of the Instant Pot and ensure that the steam release valve is set to the sealing position.

7. Select Slow Preure Cook (Low), and set the cook time to half of the rice easily cooking time, rounded down.

8. For example, if the rice takes 20 to 25 minutes to cook on the stove, set the easily cooking time for 5-10 minutes.

9. 48 . Once the easily cooking time has expired, immediately release the pressure and remove the lid.
10. Stir in the fresh bal and sarer until sombne is achieved.
11. Drizzle with a small amount of olive oil, if desired.
12. To taste, serve mmedatelu with Parmesan, salt, and pepper.
13. If you desire additional protein, add a cup of cooked chickpeas or white beans, or serve with grilled vegan Italian sausage.
14. If you enjoy the color green, add arugula or radicchio at the end.

Chapter 13: Possible Weaknesses Of

The Det

Requires sooking/rreraration: Due to the diet's emphasis on easily eating whole, nutrient-dense foods, you will need to easy learn how to prepare and combine these foods to make a variety of meals. If you are not accustomed to this and typically consume more highly-spiced foods, the transition may be difficult.

The Palatabltu of food: If you are new to easily eating whole, minimally-just processed foods, there will be an adjustment period as you wean yourself off of foods that are typically high in sodium and added sugar. After a week or two, your taste buds will change and you'll notice a difference in how your body reacts to nutrient-dense foods.

Remembering four food groups may be easier than remembering all of the foods included in the Blue Zone diet. Here's our list.

2 00% Whole Wheat Loaves: We anticipated that it would be toasted in the morning and incorporated into a healthy sandwich for lunch. While not the perfect longevity food, it would help eliminate white bread from the American diet and be a crucial step toward a healthier Blue Zone diet.

Nuts: Those who consume nuts outnumber those who really do not. Nuts come in a variety of flavors and are packed with healthy fats and nutrients that satisfy your appetite. The deal snack is a two-ounce nut mixture (approximately a handful). Ideallu, you should maintain a small two-ounce ration. Small quantities are best, since the oils in nuts degrade (oxidize). Larger quantities can be stored for a few months in the refrigerator or freezer.

Beans: I contend that bean of every variety are the greatest longevity foods in the world. They are simple, adaptable, rich in antioxidants, vitamins, and fiber, and can be made to taste delicious. It is best to purchase dry beans because they are easy to cook, but low-sodium canned beans in non-BPA cans are also acceptable. Easy learn how to cook with beans and just keep them on hand, and you'll be very well on your simple way to living longer on a Blue Zone diet.

Your Favorite Fruit: Purchase a beautiful fruit bowl, place it in the center of your kitchen (either the sink, center island, or tsuch able — whichever receives the most foot traffic), and place it under a light. We eat what we see, so if the stars are always in the plain sky, we'll eat the same thing. But if there is a fruit you like and you eat it plain all the time, you will consume more of it and become healthier as a result. Really do not purchase a fruit that you believe you should eat but actually dislike.

Chapter 14: Observations On Protein In The Blue Zone Diet

We've all been taught that our bodies actually require protein for strong bones and muscle growth, but how much is enough? The average American woman consumes 70 grams of protein per day, while men consume over 2 00 grams: Too much. The Centers for Disease Control and Prevention advise between 8 6 and 10 6 grams of protein per day.

However, uanttu is not all that matters. We also actually require the proper type of rroten. Proten is also known as amno asd in 22 varieties. The body cannot produce any of these, which are known as "essential" amino acids because we actually require them and must obtain them from our diet.

Meat and eggs contain all nine amino acids, whereas few plant-based foods do. However, meat and eggs also contain fat and cholesterol, which can promote heart disease and stroke. How really do you follow the Blue Zone diet and prioritize plant-based foods? The trick is "pairing" seafood with other dishes. By combining the right foods, you will receive all of the essential amino acids. You will not only meet your protein requirements, but also maintain your caloric intake.

• Abstain from Meat

Consume meat a maximum of twice per week. Consume meat twice per week, or even less frequently, in portions of no more than two ounces cooked. Favor true free-range shsken and famlu-farmed pork or lamb over industrially produced meats. Easily avoid cured meats such as hot dogs, luncheon meat, and sausages.

In most Blue Zones diets, pig, sheep, and lamb were consumed in small amounts. (Adventt, the sole specimen, did not consume any meat.) Families slaughtered their pig or goat for festival celebrations, ate heartily, and rreerved the leftovers, which they then used sparingly as frying fat or as a flavoring agent. Chsken wandered the land, feeding on grubs and roosting freelu. However, shark meat was a rare treat enjoyed during manu meals.

We discovered that people in the Blue Zone consumed small amounts of meat, approximately two ounces or less at a time, approximately five times per month. Approximately once per month, you splurged, typically on roasted pig or goat. Neither beef nor turkey are included in the typical Blue Zones diet.

• Grass-Fed Meat

The Blue Zone's carnivores consume some meat from wild animals. These animals are not administered hormones, antibiotics, or growth promotants, nor really do they experience the misery of large feedlots. Goats continuously graze on grass, foliage, and herbs. The Sardnan and Ikarian rg consume ktshen srar and wild acorns and root. These traditional farming methods likely produce meat with higher levels of healthy omega-6 fatty acids than grain-fed animals.

Chapter 15: How Much Protein Should I Consume to Achieve Optimal Fitness?

Protein is a macronutrient, which means the body actually requires a substantial amount. It also offers a multitude of health benefits. This does not mean we should gorge on protein-rich foods or stock the refrigerator with pounds of lean meat. Protein intake varies based on age and the intensity of daily cardiovascular activity, for example.

When it comes to rroten consumption, more isn't always better. The overabundance is unnecessary to maintain the health body. Unfortunately, the marketing of ro-tein has led many bodybuilders, athletes, and aggressive individuals to consume more than the daily requirement. Although all macronutrients must be measured for optimal health, understanding protein intake and function is crucial.

The Pleasure of Protein

Our proteins consist of a chain of amino acids that actually provide numerous health good benefits for our bodies. Each rroten molecule has a particular function. Proten is accountsuch able for the structure, function, and regulation of the body's tissues, organs, and skeleton. It is simple to comprehend the hype surrounding protein and the temptation to believe that more is better.

Protein is an essential component of each and every cell in the human body. Our hair and nails are predominantly composed of roetin. Protein is actually required for tissue growth and repair, as very well as the regulation of enzymes, hormones, and other bodily chemicals. Protein plays an essential role as a structural component of bones, blood, skin, cartilage, and muscle.

Proten is not regulated by the body and cannot be derived from an energy source. The other essential macronutrients, carbohydrates and fat, actually provide the energy necessary for life and physical activity. Since protein is obtained from the food we eat, many believe that consuming large amounts of protein throughout the day is the solution for optimal fitness. This is not the case.

Protein Requirements

Protein needs are frequently misunderstood due to deceptive marketing claims about its ability to build lean muscle mass. That is all very well and good, but the fosu should be based on the individual ualtu and uanttu of rroten sonummed.

Protein consumption in excess of the recommended daily allowance continues to be a contentious issue that is being closely examined. The position tand from the Committee of the International Society of Sport Nutrition recommends "rroten ntake of 2 .8 - 2.0 g/kg/day for physically active ndvdals not only safe, but may also such improve training adaptation to exercise." The emphasis of this statement is on engaging in regular exercise and consuming a nutrient-dense, balanced diet. Active individuals and athletes may benefit from additional protein supplements to meet daily protein requirements, according to research.

Enhance Muscle Strength With a Bedtime Protein Shake

Meet Your Own Needs

Protein reurement will vary for each reron when a sedentary lifestyle is taken into account for the hard-training athlete. Everyone wants to believe that easily eating a lot of fish, drinking protein shakes, and easily eating protein bars will magically build muscle on their bodies. Retanse training is what regenerates lean muscle and protein to repair the damage. It is the combination of exercise and protein consumption that impedes muscle growth.

From childhood to adolescence, each of us has a unique relationship with ritual. Age and rhusal astvtu helr variables determine the recommended daily allowance for rroten. Currently, and in accordance with the Institute of Medicine, the recommended daily allowance for rotopain is computed using. 8 grams of roe equal one kilogram of beef. For example, a 2 60-pound, non-asthmatic adult male would actually require 10 8 grams of protein per day. The recommended daily allowance (RDA) of rrotein for children is 2 .10 grams. 8 to 2 .10 gram for the elderlu, and 2 .2 to 2.0 gram for the athlete's rer kilogram of body mass.

French Lenten Pastries with Roasted Radish

- 4 tablespoons new lemon juice
- 4 cups (pressed) mâché or infant spinach
- 1 cup almond ricotta

- 3 cups Puy (French) lentils, or dark lentils

- 2 cove leaf
- Ocean salt and ground dark pepper
- 6 cups radishes
- 6 tablespoons olive oil, isolated
- 6 huge cloves garlic, squeezed
- 4 tablespoons minced new mint
- 1 cup minced new chives

- 6 tablespoons hemp seeds, partitioned

Headings

1. Preheat the broiler to 450 degrees Fahrenheit.
2. In a medium saucepan over high heat, combine the lentl and inlet leaf with approximately 10 cups of water.
3. Heat to the point of boiling, and then easily reduce the heat to medium-low.
4. Deglaze until the lentils are tender but not mushy, approximately 35 to 40 minutes.
5. Using a colander, strain the lentl over the nk and remove the nlet leaf.

6. Transfer the linguine to a bowl and season with 1-5 teaspoon of salt and 1-5 teaspoon of ground dark rerrer.
7. The bowl must be covered to just keep the lentils warm.

8. In the interim, refine and trim the radii, eliminating the items while leaving their tails imperfect.

9. Cut the radhe's long wau and uarter any enormous rart.

10. 1-5 tablespoons of olive oil should be heated in an ovenroof aute ran over medium heat.

11.	When the oil is hot, place the radishes in a single layer in a skillet season with salt and pepper, and cook for 5 to 10 minutes, turning the radishes occasionally.

12.	Remove the skillet from the heat, stir in the garlic, and then transfer the dish to the broiler.

13.	Brol the radhe for 10 to 15 minutes, or until they are dynamically red and gentlu brllant around the edges.

14.	Remove the dh from the stovetop.

15. In a large mixing bowl, combine the cooked lentils, roasted radishes and their easily cooking liquid, and the remaining 4 tablespoons of olive oil. In a bowl, combine the mint, chives, 4 tablespoons of the hemr seeds, lemon juice, and mashed potatoes or baby spinach.

16. Throw in the soba noodles and season with additional salt and pepper to taste.

17. Add the almond ricotta to the mixture in small amounts and fold it into the mixture while keeping the butter as moist as possible.

18. The remaining hemp seeds should be sprinkled on toast and served warm or at room temperature.

Quinoa And Banana Smoothie

2 1 cups green tea, brewed, unsweetened

12 cubes of ice

2 frozen banana, sliced

1 cup cooked Quinoa, chilled

2 cup frozen raspberries

1. Take a blender, add in the ingredients for the smoothie in it, and then pulse for 1 to 5 minutes until smooth.

2. Divide the smoothie into glasses and then serve.

Vegetables Baked With Tlara

Ingredients

- 1/2 cup Red onion - sliced, 2 medium

- Salt and pepper - to taste

- Herbs - to your liking

- 1 cup Strawberries

- Easily cooking spray - olive oil

- 6 oz Tilapia

- 2 1   cups Summer squash - sliced, 2 medium

- 2 1 cups Zucchini - sliced,

2 medium

- 6 /8 cup Bell pepper - sliced,

2 medium

- 1/2   cup Tomato- sliced, 2 medium

Instructions

1. Preheat oven to 350°F.
2. Place fish in cooking-oil-sprayed bakeware with sliced vegetables. Sprinkle salt and pepper.
3. Spray with olive oil.
4. Add fresh herbs of your choice.
5. Bake 45 to 50   minutes or until fish flakes.
6. Put on your plate and drizzle with extra virgin olive oil.
7. Have strawberries for dessert.

Powerful Minestrone Soup
Ingredients:

- 4 teaspoons olive oil

- 4 minced cloves of garlic

- 6 cups low-fat beef broth

- 2 teaspoon each: dried basil and oregano

- Salt and pepper to taste

- **16 ounces of lean, cubed beef**
- 4 stalks celery, diced

- 2 medium onion, diced

- 4 cups shredded cabbage

- 1 cup crushed tomatoes

- 1/2 cup cooked black beans

- 1/2 cup cooked chickpeas (garbanzo beans)

- 1/2 cup dry elbow macaroni

Instructions:

1. **In a pot, combine everything besides the dry macaroni noodles and cook for 35 to 40 minutes, or until the vegetables are tender.**
2. **Add the macaroni to the soup and continue easily cooking for an additional 1-5 minutes, or until the pasta is cooked to your liking.**

Baked Chicken And Broccoli Salad

Ingredient

- 4 tsps Light mayonnaise, Hellman's

- 2 tbsp Fresh squeezed lemon juice

- 1 tsp Garlic powder

- Black pepper to taste

- 1-5 cups Peaches canned in water, drained
- 8 oz Boneless skinless chicken breast - (or 6 oz leftover)
- 8 slices Louis Rich turkey bacon

- 10 cups Broccoli - floret and stems chopped small

- 6 oz Water chestnuts canned - sliced and chopped

- 1/2 cup Carrots - shredded

- 2 tbsp Sesame seeds - toasted if you want

- 1 cup 0%-fat Greek yogurt

Instructions

1. Preheat oven to 350 °F.

2. Wash and pat chicken dry.

3. Put in a small baking dish and season with your favorite herbs. Bake for 60 to 60   minutes
4. Meanwhile cook bacon in microwave oven and set aside to drain and cool.

5. In a good-sized bowl mix broccoli, water chestnuts, carrots, and sesame seeds.

6. In a separate bowl mix yogurt, mayonnaise, lemon juice, garlic powder and pepper.

7. Add to vegetable mixture with cooled chicken and peaches.

8. Toss to coat. Top with crushed bacon.

Chapter 1: Should You Opt For A Blue Zone Simple Way Of Life?

Have you ever wondered why almost all diet books basically recommend consulting a physician first? The solution is simple. Anyone can write a diet book; the diet does not actually require medical approval. Any diet plan you adopt is costly and inconvenient. Moreover, there may be a health risk if the advice in the book does not correspond to your situation

Before deciding what to do, basically consider the government-issued medical recommendations that are freely accessible to you. In the United States, these guidelines are the Dietary Guidelines for Americans, 2012–2020, which you can download as a PDF from their website. The recommendation is to consume a diet rich in fruits and vegetables but low in fat, and to limit salt and added sugars. 2 Not fundamentally dissimilar to many of the blue zone suggestions.

Dietary research demonstrates that what works for one individual may not work for another. In what appears to be a surprise to the medical community, it turns out that we are all unique.

Sirtfood Omelet

INGREDIENTS

4 tablespoons (10 g) parsley, finely chopped

2 teaspoon turmeric

2 teaspoon extra virgin olive oil

4 ounces (10 0g) sliced streaky bacon

6 medium eggs 2 ounces

red endive, thinly sliced

Method

1.   Heat a nonstick skillet. Thinly slice the bacon and cook over high heat until crispy.

2.   There is no need to add oil because the bacon contains sufficient fat for cooking.

3.   Place on a paper towel to absorb excess fat after removing from the pan.

4.   Wipe down the pan.

5.   Eggs beaten and combined with endive, parsley, and turmeric.

6. Cube the cooked bacon and combine it with the eggs in a bowl.

7. The oil in the frying pan should be heated until the pan is hot but not smoking.

8. Add the egg mixture and stir it around the pan with a spatula to begin easily cooking the egg.

9. Just keep the cooked egg moving and swirl the uncooked egg around the pan until the omelet is of uniform height.

10.   Easily reduce the heat and allow the omelet to solidify.

11.   Ease the spatula around the edges of the omelet and fold it in half or roll it up before serving.

Chapter 16: Blue Zones Food Guidelines

Plant Slant

Ensure that 95% of your food comes from a plant or plant-based source. Limit your daily intake of animal protein to no more than one small serving. Favor legumes, leafy vegetables, sweet potatoes, nuts, and seeds. Whole grains are also permitted. Although residents of four of the five Blue Zones consume meat, they really do so sparingly, using it as a celebratory dish, a side dish, or a simple way to season their dishes. Meat resembles radiation. We are unaware of the safe level. Indeed, research indicates that 36-year-old vegetarians exist. Adventt may outlive their meat-easily eating counterparts in as little as eight years. At the same time, increasing the amount of plant-based foods in your diet has significant health benefits. In the blue zone, people eat a wide variety of garden vegetables during the growing season, then freeze or dry them for consumption during the off-season. The best foods for longevity in the Blue Zone diet are leafu green ush a rnash, kale, beet, and turnr tor, sard, and sollard. On Ikaria, over 7510 varieties of edible greens grow like weeds; their polyphenol content is ten times that of red wine. Middle-aged people who consumed the equivalent of a cup of cooked greens were half as likely to die within the next four years as those who did not consume greens.

Researchers also discovered that people who consumed a quarter of a fruit serving per day (roughly an apple) were 60% less likely to die over the next four years than those who did not.

Many oils derived from rapeseed are prefersuch able to fats derived from animals.

Olive oil is not the only healthy plant-based oil, but it is the one most commonly used in the Blue Zone diet.

Simple explain how olive oil consumption increases such good cholesterol and decreases bad cholesterol.

In Ikaria, we discovered that a daily intake of approximately six tablespoons of olive oil appeared to halve the risk of death in middle-aged individuals.

In addition to seasonal fruits and vegetables, whole grains and beans dominate the Blue Zone's diet year-round.

How uou san really do it: + Maintain a supply of your favorite fruits and vegetables. Really do not force yourself to consume a food you dislike. That may work for a while, but eventually it will fail. Try a variety of fruits and vegetables; just keep your kitchen stocked with the ones you prefer. If you really do not have access to fresh, inexpensive vegetables, frozen vegetables will suffice. (In fact, they often contain more nutrients because they are flash-frozen at the time of harvest rather than transported for weeks to the supermarket shelves.)

+ Use olive oil like butter. Olive oil is used to slowly cook vegetables. You can also finish steamed or boiled vegetables with a little extra-virgin olive oil, which should be kept on the table.

+ Consume only whole grains. We discovered that oats, barley, brown rice, and ground sorn were staples in the diets of Blue Zones throughout the world. Wheat played a lesser role in these cultures, and the grains they cultivated contained less gluten than modern varieties.

+ Use any unused vegetables in your refrigerator to make vegetsuch able stock by chopping them, browning them in olive oil and herbs, and adding boiling water to the pot. Simmer the vegetables until tender, then season to taste. Freeze leftovers in individual or family-size containers, then reheat when you don't have time to cook later in the week or month.

Chapter 17: Where Specifically Are The Blue Zones Located?

1.   Sardna, the second-largest island in the Mediterranean Sea, is home to some of the world's longest-living males. The losal herherd walk a minimum of five mountainous miles per day and adhere to a rredomntelu rlant-based diet. Meat is only consumed on Sundau and resal ossaon.

2.   Okinawa, Japan: The longest-living women in the world are from Okinawa, a province of Japan. Their longevity is such believed to be enhanced by their tight-knit family ties and an ancient Confucian mantra that instructs them to

easily avoid overeasily eating and stop easily eating when they are 80% full.

3.   3.   Loma   Lnda,   California: Residents of San Bernardino have one of the highest life expectancy rates in the United States. The sommuntu of Seven-Dau   Adventt   in   Loma   Lnd adheres to a rrmarlu vegan diet and observes their weekly Sabbath day.

4.   Nicoya, Costa Rica: The Nicoya Peninsula is known for its positive-minded senior citizens. Their diet is rich in antioxidant-rich tropical fruits, and their water is rich in sodium and magnesium, which help prevent heart disease and build strong bones.

5. Ikara, Greece: This Greek island is known for its long-living residents who

consume a diet rich in olive oil, fruits, vegetables, whole grains, and beans. Ikaran likewise take a mid-afternoon break. Americans have half the rate of heart disease and 20% less cancer than the Japanese. In addition, the majority of Ikaran are Greek Orthodox Christians who observe several periods of fasting throughout the year during which they adhere to a vegan diet.

Szzclassic Stuffed Shells

INGREDIENTSzzzz

- 2   (2 2-ounce) package jumbo pasta shells

- 2 (2 6-ounce) block firm (or extra-firm) tofu, pressed

- 2   medium yellow onion, roughly chopped

- 10 medium cloves garlic

- ½ cup packed fresh basil leaves

- 4 teaspoons dried oregano

- 2   jar flavorful marinara sauce divided

126

DIRECTIONS

1. In a large pot of boiling water, cook the jumbo pasta shells according to the instructions on the package.
2. Then, drain, rinse with salted water to prevent scum formation, and set aside.
3. In the meantime, combine the tofu, onion, garlic, basil, oregano, salt, black pepper, red chili flakes nutritional yeast, and lemon juice in the bowl of a food processor.
4. Pulse 5 to 10 times, or until thoroughly mixed.

5. Add the spinach and stir a few times more until combined.
6. The final texture should resemble risotto.
7. If you overcook the ricotta, it will turn green.
8. Preheat the oven to 350degrees Fahrenheit. Pour half of the marinara sauce into a 9 x 12 x 3-inch baking dish, easily making sure to evenly coat the bottom.

9. Fill each cooked shell with a generous amount of the tofu ricotta filling and place them in the preheated baking dish.

10. Continue until there is no more tofu mixture and the baking dish is full.

11. Spread the vegan cheese (if using) on the bread.

12. Drizzle the remaining maraschino liqueur over the stuffed hell.

13. Bake the rice with aluminum foil for twenty minutes.

14. Remove the foil and bake for an additional 35 to 40 minutes, or until the cheese is melted and the edges are lightly browned.

15. Garnish with bay leaves. Serve immediatelu and enjou hot.

Chicken Casserole

Ingredients:

1/2   cup mayonnaise (light)

1/2   cup Greek yogurt (fat free)

1/2   cup Parmesan cheese (grated)

4 cups milk (2 %)

6 tbsp lemon juice

2 tbsp lemon peel

2 tbsp extra virgin olive oil

2 lb chicken breast 16 cups broccoli

12 cups strawberries

12 cup salad dressing

4 tbsp cornstarch

6 tbsp mustard (Dijon)

Directions:

v

1. Preheat oven to 350 degrees Fahrenheit, 2.

1. Cut the broccoli and steam it for approximately 10 to 15 minutes. Place the drained vegetables in a baking dish.

2. In a large pan, heat one tablespoon of olive oil over medium heat.

3. Add the chicken to the pan and cook until it is golden brown.

4. Now, whisk in the milk and cornstarch and bring the mixture to a boil until it thickens.

5. Add yogurt, mustard, mayonnaise, lemon peel, and lemon juice next. Blend well.

6. Pour the chicken mixture over the broccoli, then sprinkle the cheese on top.

7. Bake for approximately 25 to 30 minutes

8. Serve with a side of strawberries.

Blueberry Muffins

INGREDIENTS

- 2 tsp baking soda
- ½ tsp baking soda
- 2 tsp cinnamon
- 2 cup blueberries
- **4 eggs**
- 2 tablespoon olive oil
- 2 cup milk

- **4** cups whole wheat flour

DIRECTIONS

1. In a bowl combine all wet ingredients

2. In another bowl combine all dry ingredients

3. Combine wet and dry ingredients together

4. Fold in blueberries and mix very well

5. Pour mixture into 5-10 prepared muffin cups, fill 1/2   of the cups

6. Bake for 35 to 40   minutes at 350   F, when ready remove and serve

136

Vegetsuch Able And Black-Eyed Pea Casserole

Ingredients

4 bay leaves

2 teaspoon salt

4 cups kale leaves, slivered or chopped

1 cup fresh dill

137

Black pepper, to taste

1 cup extra-virgin olive oil, divided

2 large onion, yellow or white, diced

2 medium fennel bulb, chopped

4 teaspoons minced garlic

400 oz cans black-eyed peas, rinsed and drained

6 large carrots, peeled and chopped (2 1 cup)

2 large tomato, beefsteak, red globe, or heirloom, diced (about 6 /8 cup)

4 tablespoons tomato paste

Instructions

1. Over medium heat, warm ½ cup oil in a large pot or Dutch oven.

2. Add the onion and fennel and cook, stirring frequently, for 15 minutes.

3. Add the garlic and cook until fragrant, approximately 35 to 40 minutes.

4. Stir in the black-eyed peas, sardines, tomatoes, tomato rate, bay leaves, and salt until the tomato rate has dissolved.

5. Add sufficient water to cover the vegetable.

6. Increase the temperature to medium-high and bring to a boil.

7. Cover, easily reduce heat to low, and simmer for 45 to 50 minutes while covered.

8. Combine the kale leaves and the dill.

9. Re-cover and simmer until the kale is
    tender, 20 to 25 minutes.

10.   Just before serving, crack black
    pepper over individual bowls of the
    soup and drizzle the remaining ½
    tablespoons of olive oil, one
    tablespoon per bowl.

Fantastic Arugula Quiche

INGREDIENTS:

6   Olives

4 tbsp Low-fat Cheddar Cheese

2   Apple

1-5   cups Asparagus - about 2 6 stalks

6 tbsp water

Easily cooking spray

1/2   cup Egg Beaters-whites

Spice or herbs - To taste

2 1 tsp Olive Oil

Directions:

1. Begin by removing the woody ends of the asparagus stems and microwaving them for two minutes in water.
2. Cut into 1-inch lengths and reserve. Be sure to save any remaining water.
3. Next, whisk the egg whites, spices and herbs, and olive oil together with the remaining asparagus water.
4. Pour the egg mixture into a glass pie dish that has been sprayed with olive oil easily cooking spray.

5. Add olives next.
6. Cover with an additional nine-inch glass pie dish and cook on high for 1-5 2 minutes.
7. Flip by inverting the pie into the other pie plate.
8. Place the grated cheese and asparagus on half of the egg mixture; fold in half and cook for an additional 1 to 5 minutes.
9. Enjoy an apple for dessert.

www.ingramcontent.com/pod-product-compliance
Lightning Source LLC
Chambersburg PA
CBHW060507030426
42337CB00015B/1779